Table of Contents

PREVIEW 4

BULIMIA DIET RECIPES 5

BREAKFAST 5

   1. Tiella! Vegetable Casserole 5

   2. Butternut Squash Bake With Apples 7

   3. Ham And Broccoli Crustless Quiche 10

   4. Low Oxalate Vegetable Casserole 12

   5. Slow Cooker Stuffed Cabbage Rolls 15

   7. Copycat PF Chang's Lettuce Wrap Recipe 20

   8. Apple Butternut Squash Cobbler Recipe 22

   9. Old Fashioned Bread Pudding Recipe 25

   10. Double Crust Chicken Pot Pie 27

LUNCH 30

   11. Apple Rice Salad 30

   12. Chicken N' Orange Salad Sandwich 32

   13. Turkey Burgers 33

   14. Canned Fish Tacos 35

   15. Chicken and Corn Chowder 36

   16. Chicken and Dumplings 38

   17. Chinese Chicken Salad 40

   18. Cider Cream Chicken 42

   19. Cowboy Caviar Bean and Rice Salad 44

   20. Ginger-Lime Shrimp on Egg Noodles 46

DINNERS 48

21. Low Oxalate Vegetable Casserole {Tiella!} 48

22. tuna thai red curry 51

23. curried black eyed pea salad sandwiches (gluten-free, vegan).... 53

24. lentil veggie tacos 55

25. authentic vegan german potato salad (gluten-free, paleo, allergy-free) 57

26. Buffalo Tahini Quinoa & Rice Wraps 59

27. Summer kale salad 61

28. Summer veggie pasta salad 63

29. Harissa Potato Salad 65

30. Cold Italian Pasta Salad 67

SNACKS 70

31. Beef Jerky 70

32. Cornichon Pickles, Low Salt 72

33. Cornbread Muffins 74

34. Edamole Spread 76

35. Fruit Salsa 77

36. Homemade Buckaroos Recipe 78

37. Healthy Air Fryer Falafel 81

38. Baked Mini Powdered Doughnuts Copycat Hostess Donettes..... 83

39. Healthy Homemade Vegan Doritos "Nacho Cheese" Flavor (Gluten-Free, Allergy-Free)... 85

40. Mini Chickpea Flour Vegan Frittata Bites 88

PREVIEW

Bulimia (boo-LEE-me-uh) nervosa, commonly called bulimia, is a serious, potentially life-threatening eating disorder. People with bulimia may secretly binge — eating large amounts of food with a loss of control over the eating — and then purge, trying to get rid of the extra calories in an unhealthy way.

To get rid of calories and prevent weight gain, people with bulimia may use different methods. For example, you may regularly self-induce vomiting or misuse laxatives, weight-loss supplements, diuretics or enemas after bingeing. Or you may use other ways to rid yourself of calories and prevent weight gain, such as fasting, strict dieting or excessive exercise.

If you have bulimia, you're probably preoccupied with your weight and body shape. You may judge yourself severely and harshly for your self-perceived flaws. Because it's related to self-image — and not just about food — bulimia can be hard to overcome. But effective treatment can help you feel better about yourself, adopt healthier eating patterns and reverse serious complications.

BULIMIA DIET RECIPES

BREAKFAST

1. Tiella! Vegetable Casserole
Prep Time: 20 minutes

Cook Time 1 hour

Total Time: 1 hour 20 minutes

Ingredients

- Tomato sauce homemade or in a jar (if in a hurry)
- Sliced zucchini or squash or both minimum one medium zucchini
- 2 medium to large potatoes sliced 1/4 inch
- 1/4 cup Grated Parmesan cheese I use more if you are a cheese fan
- Breadcrumbs
- Salt and pepper to taste
- Optional: one small chopped onion and green peppers sliced

Instructions

1. You know how family recipes are... the amounts of the ingredients are somewhat sketchy. Judge the amount of vegetables as to the size of the dish.

2. I used an eight inch square glass dish.

3. Spritz the glass dish with cooking spray.

4. Add one layer of sliced zucchini and potatoes, (any optional vegetables), tomato sauce, sprinkle with parmesan and bread crumbs.

5. Cheese alert! I am very generous with the cheese and liberally sprinkle the cheese on each layer so I use 1/2 cup in total. A 1/4 cup of cheese per layer.

6. Repeat.

7. You can now see what this dish is also known as the layered vegetable casserole.

8. Bake at 350 degrees for approximately 50 minutes. Check the dish for doneness by inserting a fork into the vegetables. The vegetables should be fork tender.

9. As you know, potatoes take longer to cook, I baked the dish another 20 minutes. If you are worried the breadcrumbs are becoming too brown, then cover the dish with foil at the 50 minute mark.

10. Check the doneness again with the fork.

2. Butternut Squash Bake With Apples

Prep Time: 20 minutes

Cook Time: 30 minutes

Total Time: 50 minutes

Servings: 8

Ingredients

- 1 10 ounce bag of frozen butternut squash OR 1 medium butternut squash about 1.5 pounds works well
- 1 tablespoon butter
- 1/2 teaspoon salt
- 1/4 teaspoon pepper
- 3 medium apples peeled and cored or 12 oz. applesauce
- 1/4 teaspoon cinnamon
- 1 tablespoon sugar
- Need to add some crunch to the ? This is a very flexible and very forgiving side dish. A crunchy sweet topping can be added to the entire dish or just half the dish to satisfy all ! Add the topping before baking.

Topping

- 1 cup slightly crushed cornflakes
- 1/4 cup chopped pecans or the nut of your choice
- 1 tablespoon melted butter
- 1 tablespoon brown sugar
- Mix into a crumble and add to the Butternut Squash Apple Bake before baking.
- Or skip the crumble and just add your favorite nuts to the top after baking.

Instructions

1. Preheat oven to 350 degrees.
2. Microwave the butternut squash per directions on the bag. If using fresh butternut squash peel squash, remove seeds, cut into large pieces. This is the most labor intensive part of the recipe, it can be tough to tame a butternut squash, be careful! Boil squash for 20-30 minutes until tender. Drain.
3. In a medium bowl, add the butternut squash and very gently mash a few of the pieces.
4. Add remaining ingredients and gently mix. This will determine the smoothness of the dish.

5. Spoon into a 9" pie dish or an 8" square glass dish. The consistency will be fluffy!

6. Bake 25-30 minutes at 350 degrees.

7. Need to add some crunch to the ? This is a very flexible and very forgiving side dish. A crunchy sweet topping can be added to the entire dish or just half the dish to satisfy all ! Add the topping before baking.

3. Ham And Broccoli Crustless Quiche

Prep Time: 15 minutes

Cook Time: 30 minutes

Total Time: 45 minutes

Servings: 6

Ingredients

- 1 cup diced ham
- 1 cup broccoli florets frozen or fresh
- 4 eggs
- 4 egg whites
- 1/4 cup water
- 1 cup low fat cottage cheese can use regular
- Salt and pepper to taste

Instructions

1. Prepare a 9 " baking dish, pie dish or quiche dish with cooking spray.
2. Heat oven to 375 degrees.
3. Prepare your broccoli by pre cooking either in the microwave or on the stove top.

4. Dice the ham while the broccoli is cooking.

5. Using a large bowl, whisk the eggs, egg whites and water.

6. Now add the cottage cheese and whisk with intent! You want the cottage cheese to become fairly smooth and mix in with the egg mixture.

7. Pour into prepared dish. Place the broccoli and ham into the mixture.

8. Bake for 30 to 35 minutes. Check at the 30 minute mark.

4. Low Oxalate Vegetable Casserole
Prep Time: 20 minutes

Cook Time: 50 minutes

Total Time: 1 hour 10 minutes

Serving: 4

Ingredients

- 1 jar Squash sauce homemade or in store bought (if in a hurry)
- 1 each Sliced zucchini or squash (one of each) or (minimum one medium zucchini)
- 1 bag frozen Cauliflower florets can use fresh
- 1/2 cup Grated Parmesan cheese I use more if you are a cheese fan
- 1 small chopped onion
- 1 small chopped pepper
- 1 sleeve Crushed saltines 1 cup breadcrumbs
- Salt and or white pepper to taste

Instructions

1. I use either a smaller rectangle 7 X 11 " glass baking dish or an eight inch square glass dish.
2. A 13 X 9 baking dish can be used to serve a larger crowd, but the ingredients need to be increased by 25 percent(ish.) This is a very flexible dish and can be tweaked with quantity or vegetable; all work!
3. Coat the glass dish with cooking spray.
4. Add one layer of sliced zucchini or sliced zucchini and squash.
5. Add the onions and peppers and cauliflower florets on top of the zucchini layer.
6. Pour the squash sauce over the vegetables, sprinkle with parmesan and crushed saltines.
7. Cheese alert! I am very generous with the cheese and liberally sprinkle the cheese on each layer so I use 1/2 cup in total. A 1/4 cup of cheese after the zucchini layer and then on top of all the vegetables before the crunchy topping is added.
8. The layered vegetable casserole is now ready for the oven.
9. Bake at 350 degrees for approximately 50 minutes. Zucchini and squash bake quicker than the cauliflower so check the dish for doneness by inserting a fork into the vegetables. The vegetables should be fork tender.

10. If additional cooking time is necessary, I cover the dish with foil as I do not want the crunchy saltine top to over brown. I baked the dish another 20 minutes.

11. Give the vegetables another fork test for tenderness. I prefer softer vegetables, but if a firmer vegetable is preferred then baking for 50 minutes total works well.

5. Slow Cooker Stuffed Cabbage Rolls

Prep Time: 30 minutes

Cook Time: 5 hours

Total Time: 5 hour 30 minutes

Servings: 6

Equipment

Slow Cooker

Ingredients

- 1 large head of green cabbage
- 1 lb ground beef
- 1 lb lean ground pork
- 1 tbsp coconut oil
- ½ white onion diced finely
- 1-1/2 cups of rice rice does not need to be precooked
- ½ tsp garlic powder
- ½ tsp sea salt
- 1 tsp black pepper
- 8 oz crushed tomatoes
- 4 oz tomato paste

Instructions

1. In a large bowl, mix the beef, pork, garlic powder, salt and pepper.
2. Put a large pot of water on the stove over high heat. To prepare the cabbage for rolling, lightly boil it whole and peel the leaves off a few at a time. Cut the core out of the cabbage and place in the pot. Bring to a boil and then reduce the heat to a simmer. As the leaves soften, you can peel them off with a spoon or pair of tongs.
3. In a large skillet over medium-high heat, add a tablespoon of coconut oil , add the onion and sauté for 3 to 5 minutes until the onion is translucent.
4. Combine the onion and rice with the meat, and mix by hand to incorporate all the ingredients.
5. Take a cabbage leaf, concave side up with the stem toward you, and place a large spoonful of the meat mixture at the stem end.
6. Then roll forward, fold the sides in and end with the seam down.
7. Mix the crushed tomatoes and tomato sauce in a bowl. Put about 1 cup in the bottom of the slow cooker. Lay the cabbage rolls in with the seam side down. Cover with the remaining tomato mixture once the slow cooker is full.
8. Cook on low for 5 hours.

6. Aloha Hawaiian Chicken

Prep Time: N/A

Cook Time: N/A

Total Time: N/A

Servings: 6

Ingredients

- 2 pounds boneless, skinless chicken breasts
- 1 cup cornstarch
- 3 large eggs, beaten
- 1/4 cup vegetable oil
- salt and pepper, to taste

For Hawaiian Sauce:

- 1 cup pineapple juice (can also use juice from canned pineapple)
- 1/2 cup dark brown sugar
- 1/3 cup low sodium soy sauce
- 1 clove minced garlic
- 1/2 Tablespoon cornstarch

- 1 chopped red bell pepper
- 1 (20 oz.) can of pineapple tidbits. Drain the can and reserve the juice for the Hawaiian sauce

Instructions

1. Grease a 9×13-inch baking pan and preheat the oven to 325 degrees.
2. Season chicken with salt and pepper. Cut in bite-size pieces.
3. Place cornstarch in a quart size or gallon size plastic bag.
4. Place eggs in a separate medium bowl.
5. Place chicken pieces in the plastic bag filled with cornstarch. Shake to coat chicken pieces.
6. Then dip cornstarch coated chicken into the eggs.
7. Heat vegetable oil in a large, non-stick skillet over medium-high heat. Olive oil works too.
8. Cook coated and dipped chicken until golden-brown on all sides. Place chicken in the prepared dish. Do not cook chicken fully as the chicken will cook in the oven.
9. In a medium bowl whisk together the Hawaiian sauce ingredients; pineapple juice, brown sugar, low sodium soy sauce, garlic and cornstarch. Pour evenly over chicken.

10. Sprinkle the top of the chicken with the chopped bell pepper and pineapple.

11. Bake chicken uncovered for 1 hour. It is recommended to stir the chicken every 15 minutes to ensure the chicken pieces remain coated in sauce.

12. Remove from oven and let stand 5 minutes before serving.

7. Copycat PF Chang's Lettuce Wrap Recipe

Prep Time: 15 minutes

Cook Time: 5 minutes

Total Time: 15 minutes

Servings: 4

Ingredients

- 1-1.5 breasts of leftover seasoned chicken or rotisserie chicken depends upon size of chicken breast
- 1 can of water chestnuts
- 2 tablespoons low sodium soy sauce
- 2 tablespoons of brown sugar sugar substitute if watching sugar intake
- 1/2 teaspoon rice vinegar
- 1 teaspoon minced garlic
- 2 to 3 tablespoons dried chives or fresh chives
- 1 tablespoon of cooking oil or olive for stir fry
- Iceberg lettuce or white rice or rice sticks

Instructions

1. Chop the water chestnuts and chicken into dice size pieces.

2. Mix together: low sodium soy sauce sauce, brown sugar, garlic, chives and rice vinegar.

3. Heat one tablespoon of oil in a large frying pan at medium high heat.

4. Add the diced chicken and water chestnuts to the pan and then add the stir fry sauce. Cook for five five minutes on medium heat then lower to medium low heat for an additional three to five minutes.

5. Ready to serve! Use leaves of iceberg lettuce as the wrap for the traditional recipe or serve over white rice. Rice Sticks are optional for oxalate friendly guests; however rice flour which is the main ingredient in rice sticks are high on the oxalate list.

8. Apple Butternut Squash Cobbler Recipe
Prep Time: 10 minutes

Cook Time: 40 minutes

Total Time: 50 minutes

Servings: 4

Ingredients

- 1 tbsp. butter
- 1/2 tbsp. Steviva Blend
- 1/2 tsp. salt
- 1/4 tsp. cinnamon
- 2 tbsp. tapioca flour

Topping

- 1 cup gluten free cornflakes
- 1/4 cup nuts
- 1 tbsp. melted butter
- 1/2 tbsp. Steviva Blend

Instructions

1. Microwave or cook the butternut squash according to the directions on the package.
2. Drain excess water from the butternut squash.
3. Cut the apples into bite size pieces.
4. TIP! For uniformity in baking cut the apples pieces to the size of the butternut squash pieces.
5. In a medium bowl combine the butternut squash, apples, butter, cinnamon, salt, tapioca flour and Stevia Blend.
6. Gently mix all ingredients.
7. Grease a 1 1/2 quart baking dish.
8. Spoon the Apple Butternut Squash Cobbler into the dish.
9. Bake at 350 degrees for 20 minutes.

While the cobbler is baking prepare the topping.

1. Melt the butter and add the cornflakes, nuts and Steviva Blend.
2. Mix the topping ingredients. Gently use the back of the spoon to crush the cornflakes. I crush about 1/2 of the cornflakes which creates a nice mixture, but it is personal preference.

3. After the cobbler has baked for 20 minutes add the topping and bake an additional 20 minutes for a total baking time of 40 minutes for the cobbler.

4. Remove from oven and serve warm.

9. Old Fashioned Bread Pudding Recipe

Prep Time: 30 minutes

Cook Time: 30 minutes

Total Time: 1 hour

Servings: 6

Ingredients

- 1 loaf of bread your choice of bread, French bread works well
- 6 eggs
- 3/4 cup sugar
- 1/4 tsp salt
- 1/2 tsp vanilla extract
- 4 cups milk
- Sprinkle lemon zest
- 1 cup raisins optional

Instructions

1. Butter a 9 by 9 inch pan, sprinkle raisins on bottom of pan.

2. Butter slices of bread, cut slices in half and lay on bottom of the pan.

3. Whisk together eggs, salt, sugar, vanilla extract, milk and lemon rind.

4. Pour over bread.

5. Place pan in a water bath.

6. Bake at 400 degrees, 20-25 minutes until set. (I found it takes 30 minutes in my oven)

10. Double Crust Chicken Pot Pie

Prep Time: 20 minutes

Cook Time: 1hour

Total Time: 1 hour 20 minutes

Serving: 4

Ingredients

- 6 boneless chicken breasts cut into 1 inch pieces
- 1 medium onion chopped
- 2 tablespoons butter melted
- 1 stalk celery chopped
- 1 ½ cups frozen mixed vegetables or fresh
- 1 cup sliced mushrooms optional
- 1 cup diced potato peeled if you are a tater lover, add more!
- 1 cup chicken broth
- ½ cup dry white wine see below for non alcohol substitutions
- ½ teaspoon dried parsley
- ¼ teaspoon pepper
- 1 bay leaf

- 2 tablespoons cornstarch
- 2 tablespoons water
- 1 10 3/4 ounce an of cream of mushroom soup, undiluted
- 1 cup 4 oz shredded cheddar cheese
- ¼ cup sour cream
- Pie Pastry of your choice store bought or homemade
- 1 egg yolk lightly beaten
- 1 tablespoon milk

Instructions

How To Make Pot Pie Filling

1. Add two tablespoons of butter to a large skillet on medium high heat. Cook chicken and onion in butter until chicken is browned and the onion is tender.
2. Stir in celery, mixed vegetables, mushroom (optional), diced potato, chicken broth, white wine, parsley, pepper and bay leaf.

3. Bring ingredients in the skillet to a boil. Cover and reduce heat.

4. Simmer 15 minutes or until vegetables are tender.

5. Discard the bay leaf.

6. Mix cornstarch and 2 tablespoons of cold water. Stir until smooth.

7. Now add the water & cornstarch to the ingredients in the skillet. Bring to a boil over medium heat and stir constantly.

8. Remove from heat and stir in the undiluted soup, cheese and sour cream.

9. Roll half of pot pie pastry and fit into an ungreased pie pan or casserole dish.

10. Spoon chicken mixture into the dish.

11. Place remaining pastry over chicken mixture. Trim edges of pie pastry, seal and crimp edges. Cut slits into top of pastry .

12. Combine the egg yolk and 1 tablespoon milk and lightly brush over pastry top.

13. Protect the edges of pastry with aluminum foil to prevent singing the pot pie pastry edges.

14. Bake at 400 degrees for 35 minutes or until golden brown.

LUNCH

11. Apple Rice Salad

Ingredients

Based on: 4 servings

- 2 tablespoons balsamic vinegar
- 1 tablespoon olive oil
- 2 teaspoons honey
- 2 teaspoons brown or dijon mustard
- 1 tablespoon orange peel, finely shredded
- 1/4 teaspoon garlic powder
- 2 cups cooked rice (any kind), chilled
- 2 cups (about 2 medium) apples, chopped
- 1 cup celery, thinly sliced
- 2 tablespoons unsalted sunflower seeds, shelled

Instructions

1. In a small bowl, combine the vinegar, olive oil, honey, mustard, orange peel, and garlic powder. Mix well and set aside.

2. In a large bowl, combine rice, apples, celery, and sunflower seeds. Toss until well mixed.

3. Drizzle the dressing over the rice salad mixture and toss until salad is well coated.

4. Serve immediately or cover and refrigerate for up to 24 hours.

12. Chicken N' Orange Salad Sandwich

Ingredients

Based on 6 servings

- 1 cup chopped cooked chicken
- 1/2 cup celery, diced
- 1/2 cup green pepper, chopped
- 1/4 cup onion, finely sliced
- 1 cup Mandarin oranges
- 1/3 cup mayonnaise

Instructions

1. Toss chicken, celery, green pepper, and onion to mix.

2. Add mandarin oranges and mayonnaise.

3. Mix gently.

4. Serve on bread.

13. Turkey Burgers
Ingredients

Based on: 4 servings

- 1 pound lean ground turkey
- 1 cup (about 3 small) zucchini, grated
- 1 large egg
- 1/4 cup panko bread crumbs
- 1/4 cup red onion, grated
- 1 each garlic clove
- 1 teaspoon salt free seasoning
- 1/2 teaspoon black pepper
- 1 tablespoon vegetable oil

Instruction

1. In a large bowl, combine all ingredients. Mix well.

2. Form equal sized patties, about half inch thick.

3. In a large non-stick skillet, heat 1 teaspoon vegetable oil on medium high heat.

4. Add patties and reduce heat to low until browned, about 5 minutes each side.

5. Make sure patties are cooked through, no longer pink in the middle.

6. Freeze extras for a quick meal later.

14. Canned Fish Tacos

Ingredients

Based on 2 servings

- 2 tablespoons chopped onion
- 2 teaspoons oil
- 1 can tuna, drained and rinsed
- 1/2 cup corn, canned or frozen
- 1/4 cup canned diced tomatoes, no salt added
- 1/2 teaspoon chili powder
- 4 corn tortillas

Instruction

1. In a frying pan cook onions in oil over medium heat until they turn clear.

2. Add tuna, corn, tomatoes, and chili powder.

3. Cook until heated through, about 3-5 minutes.

4. Serve with warm tortillas. Add sour cream, lettuce, and hot sauce if desired.

15. Chicken and Corn Chowder

Ingredients

Based on 12 servings

- 12 slices bacon, low sodium
- 2 onions, chopped
- 7 cups chicken broth, low sodium
- 4 potatoes, diced and soaked
- 8 cups Corn
- 8 boneless chicken breasts, diced
- 6 tablespoons fresh thyme, chopped
- 4 cups Mocha Mix
- 1/2 teaspoon black pepper
- 8 green onions, chopped

Instruction

1. in a pan until crisp, remove bacon and set aside.

2. Saute onions in the bacon fat.

3. Add broth and potatoes.

4. Cover and simmer for 10 mins.

5. Add corn, chicken and thyme.

6. Cover and simmer until chicken is cooked (15 mins).

7. Stir Mocha Mix into the soup and simmer 2 mins.

8. Sprinkle in bacon, pepper and green onions.

16. Chicken and Dumplings

Ingredients

Based on: 8 servings

- 1 whole chicken or 3 lbs chopped chicken
- 2 cups water or low sodium chicken broth
- 1 stalk celery with leaves, cut fine
- 2-3 carrots, sliced
- 1/2 teaspoon black pepper
- 1/2 teaspoon mace or nutmeg
- 1/4 cup flour
- 2 eggs
- 2/3 cup milk
- 3 teaspoons baking powder
- 2 cups flour
- 2 tablespoons unsalted butter or margarine

Instruction

1. Put chicken, vegetables, spices and water or broth into slow cooker.

2. Add more water, enough to cover chicken by about 1.

3. Turn cooker on low for about 6-8 hours.

4. Remove the chicken to an ovenproof dish.

5. Remove the bones if you want, they may just fall off.

6. Cover and keep warm.

7. Turn slow cooker up to high heat. Add the 1/4 cup flour and whisk quickly, to avoid lumps.

8. Cut the butter into the 2 cups of flour with two knives, a pastry cutter or food processor.

9. Blend in wet ingredients to a stiff dough and drop by spoonfuls into the boiling broth.

10. Cover the cooker, reduce the heat to prevent boiling, and cook for 15 minutes without removing the lid.

11. Put chicken in large serving dish and pour thickened sauce over, serve with dumplings.

17. Chinese Chicken Salad
Ingredients

Based on: 8 servings

- 2 packages ramen noodles
- 3 tablespoons, divided olive oil
- 2 tablespoons sesame seeds
- 2 cups cooked chicken or turkey, diced
- 1/2 head cabbage, shredded and chopped
- 4 green onions, diced
- 1/4 cup sugar or Splenda
- 1 tablespoon sesame oil
- 1/2 cup white wine vinegar or rice vinegar

Instruction

1. Take the ramen noodles and smash while still in the packet.

2. Open packages and remove the seasoning packets.

3. Heat 1 tablespoon olive oil in a skillet.

4. Add in the dry noodles and sesame seeds.

5. Toast until golden brown.

6. Mix chicken or turkey, cabbage, and green onions in a bowl, then add the ramen noodles and sesame seeds.

7. Blend sugar, sesame oil, 2 tablespoons olive oil, and vinegar in a separate bowl.

8. Dress the salad with the dressing.

18. Cider Cream Chicken
Ingredients

Based on 8 servings

- 4 bone-in chicken breasts
- 2 tablespoons unsalted butter
- 3/4 cup apple cider
- 1/2 cup half and half

Instructions

1. Melt butter over medium-high heat. Add chicken and brown on both sides.

2. Add cider and reduce heat to medium; simmer for about 20 minutes.

3. Remove chicken from skillet.

4. Boil cider until reduced to about 1/4 cup.

5. Add half and half over heat; whisk until slightly thickened.

6. Pour cream sauce over chicken and serve.

43

19. Cowboy Caviar Bean and Rice Salad
Ingredients

Based on 6 servings

- 1/2 cup fresh or frozen corn, cooked
- 3 cups rice, cooked
- 1/4 cup lime juice
- 1/2 cup olive or canola oil
- 2 tablespoons brown sugar
- 1 tablespoon Dijon mustard
- 1/2 teaspoon black pepper
- 1/2 cup red bell pepper, diced
- 1/2 cup low sodium canned black beans, drained and rinsed
- 1 jalapeño, seeded and diced
- 1/2 cup cilantro, chopped

Instructions

1. Prepare rice and corn, let cool.

2. To make the dressing whisk lime juice, oil, brown sugar, mustard, and black pepper together.

3. In a large bowl combine all other ingredients.

4. Pour dressing over salad and stir.

5. Chill for one hour in refrigerator.

20. Ginger-Lime Shrimp on Egg Noodles
Ingredients

- 6 Shrimp, (36 grams) (large, fresh), peeled, tail-on
- 2 Tbsp Ginger, chopped
- 1 Tbsp Garlic, chopped
- 2 Limes, juiced, zested
- 2 Tbsp Honey
- 2 Tbsp Cilantro, chopped
- 4 oz. Egg noodles
- 2 oz.Carrots, peeled, sliced
- 1 oz.Red onion, sliced
- 1 Tsp Sesame oil
- 1 Tsp Peanut butter (unsalted)
- 1 Tsp Sriracha sauce (Asian hot sauce with garlic)
- 1 Tbsp Chicken stock, no salt added
- ½ Cup water

Instructions

1. Combine ginger, garlic, lime juice and zest, honey, cilantro, sesame oil, peanut butter, water and Sriracha sauce together. Reserve 3 Tbsp.

2. Marinate shrimp for 25 minutes in fridge.

3. While shrimp are in fridge, place a pot of water on high, once boiling add egg noodles, cook until tender. Remove noodles from pot and place in bowl.

4. Remove shrimp from marinade, and grill for 1-2 minutes on each side. Have the chicken stock boiling.

5. Toss the noodles in the reserved marinade and place shrimp on top. Garnish with shredded carrots and red onion for an added crunch and cilantro.

6. Pour hot stock over and garnish with cilantro.

DINNERS

21. Low Oxalate Vegetable Casserole {Tiella!}
Prep Time: 20 minutes

Cook Time: 50 minutes

Total Time: 1 hour 10 minutes

Servings: 4

Ingredients

- 1 jar Squash sauce homemade or in store bought (if in a hurry)
- 1 each Sliced zucchini or squash (one of each) or (minimum one medium zucchini)
- 1 bag frozen Cauliflower florets can use fresh
- 1/2 cup Grated Parmesan cheese I use more if you are a cheese fan
- 1 small chopped onion
- 1 small chopped pepper
- 1 sleeve Crushed saltines 1 cup breadcrumbs
- Salt and or white pepper to taste

Instructions

1. I use either a smaller rectangle 7 X 11 " glass baking dish or an eight inch square glass dish.

2. A 13 X 9 baking dish can be used to serve a larger crowd, but the ingredients need to be increased by 25 percent(ish.) This is a very flexible dish and can be tweaked with quantity or vegetable; all work!

3. Coat the glass dish with cooking spray.

4. Add one layer of sliced zucchini or sliced zucchini and squash.

5. Add the onions and peppers and cauliflower florets on top of the zucchini layer.

6. Pour the squash sauce over the vegetables, sprinkle with parmesan and crushed saltines.

7. Cheese alert! I am very generous with the cheese and liberally sprinkle the cheese on each layer so I use 1/2 cup in total. A 1/4 cup of cheese after the zucchini layer and then on top of all the vegetables before the crunchy topping is added.

8. The layered vegetable casserole is now ready for the oven.

9. Bake at 350 degrees for approximately 50 minutes. Zucchini and squash bake quicker than the cauliflower so check the dish for doneness by inserting a fork into the vegetables. The vegetables should be fork tender.

10. If additional cooking time is necessary, I cover the dish with foil as I do not want the crunchy saltine top to over brown. I baked the dish another 20 minutes.

11. Give the vegetables another fork test for tenderness. I prefer softer vegetables, but if a firmer vegetable is preferred then baking for 50 minutes total works well.

22. tuna thai red curry
Servings: 2

Ingredients

- Curry:
- 1 Cup Snow Peas
- 8 Baby Corn Cobs
- 3 TB Chopped Scallions (plus more for topping)
- 1 Cup Sliced Bell Peppers (I used a mix of colors)
- 1 Cup Chopped Broccoli
- ¼ Cup Chopped Cilantro
- 1 TB Chopped Thai Basil
- 1 Tsp Minced Garlic
- ½ Tsp Ground Ginger
- 1 TB Authentic Red Curry Paste
- ¼ Cup Lite Culinary Coconut Milk
- Zest of 1 Lime
- 1 TB Lime Juice
- 1 Can Bumble Bee Prime Fillet Solid White Albacore in Water
- Cauliflower Rice:
- 2 Cups of Riced Cauliflower

- ¼ Cup Lite Culinary Coconut Milk

Instructions

1. In a large saute pan, combine all the chopped and prepped veggies with the spices, curry paste, and ¼ cup of coconut milk. Stir over medium heat for about 10 minutes until the veggies begin to soften.
2. In another pan, simple heat the riced cauliflower and ¼ cup of coconut milk for 5 minutes, just until warm and the milk is absorbed.
3. Next, you can add your can of tuna (mashed) to the vegetables still in the pan directly, or just add it, (room temperature) when you plate.
4. To plate, first add the cauliflower rice, then tuna and curried veggies. Top with additional chopped scallion and you're ready to dig in!

23. curried black eyed pea salad sandwiches (gluten-free, vegan)

Prep Time: 10 minutes

Cook Time: 10 minutes

Total Time: 20 minutes

Serving: 4

Ingredients

- 2 Cups (1 15oz Can) No-Salt Added Black Eyed Peas
- 1 Cup Chopped Celery
- 1 Cup Chopped Carrot
- ½ Cup Halved Red Grapes
- ½ Cup Unsweetened Plain Coconut Yogurt
- ¼ Cup Chopped Fresh Parsley
- 1 TB Diced Shallot
- 1 TB Nutritional Yeast
- 1 Tsp Curry Powder
- 1 Tsp Dijon Mustard
- 1 Tsp Lemon Juice
- ½ Tsp Turmeric
- ½ Tsp Paprika

- ¼ Tsp Black Pepper
- Sandwich Options:
- 4 Gluten-Free Buns
- 8 Slices of Gluten-Free Bread
- 4 Gluten-Free Wraps

Instructions

1. In a large bowl, combine all the prepared ingredients and mix well to coat and combine.
2. Chill the salad in the fridge for a few hours before serving as a side dish or sandwiches.

24. lentil veggie tacos
Servings: 4

Ingredients

- ½ Cup Uncooked Brown Lentils
- 1 Small Red Bell Pepper (chopped)
- 2 Celery Hearts (chopped)
- 1 ½ Cups Baby Portobella Mushrooms (chopped)
- ½ Cup Shredded Carrots
- 3 Handfuls of Baby Spinach
- ½ TB Chili Powder
- ½ TB Dried Cilantro
- 1 Tsp Smoked Paprika
- ½ Tsp Cumin
- ½ Tsp Onion Powder
- ½ Tsp Garlic Powder
- ¼ Tsp Cayenne
- 6 Small White Corn Tortillas

Instructions

1. Begin to cook the lentils according to package directions.

2. Meanwhile, chop the veggies.

3. After the lentils have been cooking for 15 minutes, mash them and add the prepped veggies and spices.

4. Cook the lentils and veggies together for the remainder of the cooking time or until all water is absorbed.

5. For the tortillas, warm in a preheated oven at 450°F for about 10 minutes.

6. To serve, spoon on the lentil veggie mixture to your liking and enjoy!

25. authentic vegan german potato salad (gluten-free, paleo, allergy-free)
Prep Time: 5 minutes

Cook Time: 10 minutes

Total Time: 15 minutes

Servings: 4

Ingredients

- 4 Cups (2lbs) Cubed Red Potatoes (steamed or boiled)
- ¼ Cup Minced Shallots
- ¼ Cup Homemade Coconut Bacon (or storebought)
- ¼ Cup Fresh Chopped Parsley

Vinaigrette:

- ½ Cup White Vinegar
- 1 TB Pickles Juice
- 2 Tsp Erythritol (or preferred granulated sweetener)
- 1 Tsp Whole Grain Dijon Mustard
- ½ Tsp Smoked Paprika
- ½ Tsp Black Pepper

- Salt (to taste)

Instructions

1. Cube your potatoes and boil or steam them until fork tender.
2. In a bowl, whisk together the vinaigrette ingredients.
3. In a skillet, add your minced shallots and the whisked together vinaigrette, over medium heat.
4. Allow things to saute for about 5 minutes and remove from heat.
5. Place the cooked potatoes in a large bowl, add the vinaigrette, parsley, and coconut bacon. Toss together.
6. Serve right away as a warm dish or allow everything to cool before storing in a closed container in the fridge to chill.

26. Buffalo Tahini Quinoa & Rice Wraps

Cook Time: 5 mins

Total Time: 5 minus

Ingredients

- Per 1 Wrap:
- 1 Gluten-Free Wrap/Tortilla
- 1 Minute Ready To Serve Red Quinoa & Brown Rice with Garlic Cup
- 3 Romaine Leaves (sliced lengthwise)
- 1-2 Whole Carrots (sliced lengthwise)
- Buffalo Tahini Spread:
- 2 TB Tahini
- 2 Tsp Frank's Buffalo Sauce

Instructions

1. Microwave the Minute Ready To Serve Red Quinoa & Brown Rice with Garlic Cup according to package directions.
2. In a small bowl mix together the tahini and buffalo sauce until combined.

3. Lay the wrap on a plate and spread the buffalo tahini mixture over the wrap.

4. On one side of the wrap, layer on the entire quinoa and rice cup, then all the romaine and carrots.

5. Tightly roll up the wrap (like sushi). You can either wrap the rolled up wrap in plastic wrap for transport, foil for freezing, or just devour on the spot!

27. Summer kale salad
Servings: 6-8

Ingredients

- 6 Heaping Cups of Torn Curly Kale
- 1 Large Zucchini (sliced and halved)
- 1 Large Vine Ripe Tomato (chopped)
- 1 ½ Cups Snow Peas (chopped)
- 2 Scallions (green and white parts, chopped)
- Zest of 1 Small Lemon
- Juice of 1 Small Lemon
- 2 TB Chopped Fresh Parsley
- ½ Tsp Garlic Powder
- ¼ Tsp Onion Powder
- ¼ Tsp Black Pepper

Instructions

1. Prepare all you veggies and set aside. Then in a very large bowl add the kale, lemon zest and juice, garlic, onion, and pepper. Massage that baby till those

flavors are in the kale and the kale turns a darker color. You'll know when it's good!

2. Now add in all the other veggies, give everything another toss until everything is mingled. The refrigerate overnight or at least 4 hours until serving!

28. Summer veggie pasta salad
Servings: 6

Ingredients

- 8 oz (1 bag) TruRoots Gluten-Free Ancient Grain Fusilli
- 1 Small Cucumber (chopped)
- 1 Small Green Bell Pepper (chopped)
- 1 Medium Vine Ripe Tomato (chopped)
- 1 Small Red Onion (diced)
- 1 Cup Diced White Mushrooms
- 1 Cup Sweet Yellow Corn
- 1 Cup Chopped Broccoli
- ½ Cup Sliced Black Olives (rinsed)
- 1 Tsp Lemon Zest
- 2 TB Fresh Italian Parsley (chopped)
- Italian Dressing:
- ¾ Tsp Dried Oregano
- ½ Tsp Dried Basil
- ¼ Tsp Crushed Dried Rosemary
- ¼ Tsp Dried Marjoram
- ¼ Tsp Dried Thyme
- ¼ Tsp Ground Sage (scant)
- ¼ Tsp Black Pepper

- ½ Tsp Minced Garlic
- 1 TB Lemon Juice
- ½ Cup Red Wine Vinegar

Instructions

1. Cook pasta according to directions. I did the full 8 minutes. Then drain the pasta, but DO NOT rinse it. Simply set it aside in a colander while you prep your veggies.
2. In a very large mixing bowl, combine the pasta, all veggies, lemon zest, and parsley.
3. In a small bowl, combine the spices and herbs and whisk together with the vinegar and lemon juice.
4. Pour the dressing over the pasta salad and stir everything to combine and get coated.
5. Serve right away at room temperature, or refrigerate for later. Pasta salad should be served room temperature, not freezing cold, not warm and hot, but just so. Enjoy!

29. Harissa Potato Salad

Prep Time: 15 minutes

Cook Time: 40 minutes

Total Time: 55 minutes

Servings: 4

Ingredients

- 3 ½ (heaping) Cups Japanese Sweet Potatoes (about 2 small, cubed)
- 2 (heaping) Cups Red Skin Potatoes (2 small, cubed)
- 2 (heaping) Cups Broccoli (chopped, include stems)
- 2 (heaping) Cups Baby Round Eggplant
- ½ Tsp Garlic Powder
- ½ Tsp Onion Powder
- For The Sauce:
- ¼ Cup Fresh Parsley (chopped)
- ¼ Cup Carrot Top Greens (chopped)
- ¼ Cup Mina Mild Harissa*
- ½ Tsp Smoked Paprika
- ¼ Tsp Cumin
- ¼ Tsp Coriander

Instructions

1. Preheat the oven to 450°F.

2. Chop all your roasting veggies and spread out on
   a Silpat or parchment paper lined baking sheet.

3. Bake for 40 minutes, tossing everything halfway
   through.

4. To make the sauce, chop the parsley and carrot top
   greens, add to a bowl, then add in the harissa and
   spices. Give it all a mix to combine.

5. Once the veggies are finished, allow them to cool a bit
   before adding them to a large bowl and then pouring
   in the sauce. Give it all a mix and allow the flavors to
   infuse before serving warm.

30. Cold Italian Pasta Salad
Prep Time: 10 minutes

Cook Time: 10 minutes

Total Time: 20 minutes

Servings: 6-8

Ingredients

- 12 oz Gluten-Free Tri-Color Rotini*
- 2 Cups Chopped English Cucumber (1 large cucumber)
- 2 Cups Chopped Red Bell Pepper (1 medium pepper)
- 2 Cups Chopped Orange Bell Pepper (1 medium pepper)
- 2 Cups Chopped Yellow Bell Pepper (1 medium pepper)
- 2 Cups Halved Grape Tomatoes (1 pint)
- 1 Cup Chopped Red Onion (about ½ medium onion)
- 1 Cup Sliced Black Olives (1 3.8 oz can)

Italian Dressing:

- ½ Cup Extra Virgin Olive Oil

- ½ Cup Red Wine Vinegar
- 1 TB Dried Parsley
- 1 TB Dried Oregano
- 2 Tsp Dried Basil
- ½ Tsp Black Pepper

Instructions

1. Boil the gluten-free rotini according to package directions, minus about 2 minutes to keep the noodles from getting mushy.

2. In the meantime, chop the bell peppers, cucumber, tomatoes, onion, and toss them into a large bowl with the sliced black olives.

3. Drain and rinse the pasta under cold water to stop the cooking process before adding them to the chopped veggies.

4. Measure and add the olive oil, vinegar, and seasonings to the pasta salad bowl.

5. Gently mix and toss everything together in the bowl to combine.

6. Let the pasta salad marinate and chill in the fridge, for at least 30 minutes (preferably overnight), before serving.

7. Enjoy cool, at room temperature.

SNACKS

31. Beef Jerky

Ingredients

Based on 30 servings

- 3 pounds flank steak or other lean meat
- 3/4 cup sodium reduced (lite) soy sauce
- 1/2 cup red wine
- 1/4 cup dark brown sugar
- 2 tablespoons liquid smoke
- 1 1/2 teaspoons Worcestershire sauce
- 2-3 drops Tabasco sauce
- 1 teaspoon garlic powder
- 1 teaspoon liquid pepper sauce

Instructions

1. Trim (or have the butcher trim) all fat from a 3 pound flank steak or any lean meat.

2. Cut lengthwise, with the grain, into 30 long strips.

3. Place the strips in a glass dish. mix all other ingredients together and pour over the beef.

4. Cover and refrigerate for at least 5 hours or overnight.

5. When you are ready to dry the meat, remove it from the marinade.

6. If you have a dehydrator, set it for 145 degrees and dry the meat for 5-20 hours.

7. If you are using the oven, preheat to 175 degrees.

8. Put wire racks on top of baking sheets and lay the strips so they are not overlapping .

9. Bake for 10-12 hours. The beef jerky should be dry and somewhat brittle when done.

10. Store your jerky in an airtight container or plastic bag. If you are keeping it for longer than a week, store it in the freezer.

32. Cornichon Pickles, Low Salt

Ingredients

Based on 24 servings

- 3 cups cornichon or pickling cucumbers
- 1 tablespoon kosher salt
- 4 sprigs fresh tarragon
- 1/2 teaspoon mustard seeds
- enough to cover at least 1 inch above cucumbers white wine vinegar

Instructions

1. Wash the cucumbers thoroughly; drain or pat dry.

2. If small, leave the cucumbers whole. If they are bigger than your thumb then cut them in half lengthwise.

3. Place in ceramic bowl and mix well with the salt.

4. Let sit for 24 hours (does not need to be in the refrigerator).

5. Rinse quickly, drain the juices and dry the cucumbers.

6. Either put directly into jars, filling three-quarters full,
    or place into one large glass jar or crock, leaving a 2-
    inch space between the cucumbers and the top of the
    container.

7. Add the tarragon and the mustard seeds.

8. Top with white wine vinegar extending at least 1-inch
    above the cucumbers.

9. Cover jars and leave in a cool place for 3-4 weeks.

33. Cornbread Muffins

Ingredients

Based on 12 servings

- 1 cup all-purpose flour
- 1 cup cornmeal
- 1/2 teaspoon baking soda
- 1/4 cup granulated sugar
- 1/2 cup unsalted butter, softened
- 2 eggs
- 1/4 cup honey
- 1/2 cup buttermilk
- 1/2 cup no salt added canned corn

Instructions

1. Preheat oven to 400 degrees.

2. Use cooking oil spray to lightly grease a muffin pan.

3. In a large bowl, combine flour, cornmeal, baking soda and sugar.

4. Mix in butter using a pastry blender or mix in a food processor until butter is pea-sized.

5. In a separate bowl, beat eggs.

6. Mix in honey and buttermilk.

7. Pour egg mixture into the flour mixture stirring until just mixed.

8. Fold in the corn.

9. Spoon batter into muffin cups and bake for 20-25 minutes or until a toothpick inserted into the center of a muffin comes out clean.

34. Edamole Spread

Ingredients

Based on 6 (2 1/2 tablespoons each) servings

- 3/4 cup frozen shelled green soy beans (edamame), thawed
- 3 tablespoons water
- 2 tablespoons olive oil
- 1 tablespoon lemon rind, grated finely
- 1 tablespoon lemon juice
- 1/4 cup parsley leaves
- 1/4 teaspoon tabasco or hot sauce (optional)
- 1 garlic clove, halved

Instructions

1. Combine all ingredients in a food processor or blender and process until smooth.

2. Cover and chill.

3. Serve with tortilla chips or pita wedges.

35. Fruit Salsa

Ingredients

Based on 4 servings

- 3/4 cup pineapple, diced
- 3/4 cup mango, diced
- 1/2 cup strawberries, diced
- 1/4 cup red onion, diced
- 1 jalapeño, stemmed, seeded, and finely diced
- 2 tablespoons fresh mint leaves, chopped
- 2 tablespoons orange juice
- 1 tablespoon lime juice

Instructions

1. In a medium ceramic or glass bowl, combine all the ingredients and stir to blend.

2. Cover with plastic wrap and allow the salsa to marinade for 20-30 minutes before serving.

36. Homemade Buckaroos Recipe

Prep Time: 30 mins

Cook Time: 7 mins

Total Time: 37 mins

Servings: 60 cookies

Ingredients

Cinnamon graham cookies:

- ½ Cup Gluten-Free All-Purpose Flour
- ½ Cup Brown Rice Flour
- ¼ Cup Brown Sugar Erythritol (or preferred light brown sugar)
- ½ Tsp Baking Soda
- ½ Tsp Baking Powder
- ½ Tsp Cinnamon
- ½ Tsp Pure Madagascar Bourbon Vanilla Extract
- 2 TB + 1 Tsp Unsweetened Applesauce
- 2 TB Vegan/Soy-Free Butter (cold, diced)

Rainbow vanilla frosting:

- 1 Stick Vegan/Soy-Free Butter (softened)

- 2 Cups Powdered Erythritol (or preferred powdered sugar)
- 1 Tsp Pure Madagascar Bourbon Vanilla Extract
- 2 TB Unsweetened Vanilla Non-Dairy Yogurt (or a Full Fat Non-Dairy Milk)
- 2 TB Allergy-Free Rainbow Confetti Sprinkles

Instructions

For the cookies:

1. In a large mixing bowl, combine all ingredients except the applesauce and butter. Mix together.
2. Now add the applesauce and diced butter. Mix and knead the cookie dough using your hands.
3. Refrigerate the cookie dough for 30 minutes to chill and preheat the oven to 350°F in the meantime.
4. On a floured flat surface, rolling the chilled dough out to about ⅛-inch thickness. Sprinkle extra flour on the dough when rolling, if needed.
5. Cut our as many 1 inch sized cookies as you can with the dough, re-rolling as needed. I got 60 cookies using this cookie cutter.

6. Evenly space the cookies out on a Silpat or parchment paper lined baking sheet and bake the cookies for 7-8 minutes in the preheated oven.

7. Remove and let cool.

For the vanilla frosting:

1. In a stand mixer or in a bowl using a hand mixer, cream together the softened butter and powdered sugar until you get a frosting texture.

2. Next add in the vanilla extract and vanilla yogurt and blend to combine.

3. By hand fold in the rainbow sprinkles.

4. Chill the frosting in the fridge before serving.

37. Healthy Air Fryer Falafel

Prep Time: 10 mins

Cook Time: 10 mins

Total Time: 20 mins

Servings: 14 mins

Ingredients

- 2 (15oz) Cans of Chickpeas (about 3 cups)
- ½ Cup Fresh Chopped Parsley
- ½ Cup Frech Chopped Cilantro
- ½ Cup Chopped Onion
- ¼ Cup Chickpea Flour
- 1 Tsp Baking Powder
- 1 Tsp Minced Garlic
- 1 Tsp Ground Cumin
- ½ Tsp Coriander (optional)
- ½ Tsp Paprika (smoked or sweet)
- Juice of 1 Small Lemon (about 2-3 TB)

Instructions

1. In a large food processor or blender, combine all ingredients except the lemon juice.

2. Blend the mixture together to combine, adding the lemon juice, as needed, to get the mixture moving. Blend until you get a course dough.

3. Form about 14 falafel patties and work in batches to air fry, depending on the size of your air fryer basket. Do not overcrowd.

4. Air fry the falafel at 380° for about 7 minutes on the first side, flip, and air fry again for about another 5 minutes. Repeat for the rest of the batches.

5. To Bake: Preheat the oven to 400°F and bake for about 15 minutes on each side using a parchment paper or a Silpat lined baking sheet.

38. Baked Mini Powdered Doughnuts Copycat Hostess Donettes

Prep Time: 5 mins

Cook Time: 8 mins

Total Time: 13 mins

Servings: 32

Ingredients

- 1 Cup Coconut Flour
- ¼ Cup Arrowroot Starch
- 1 Tsp Baking Powder
- ½ Cup Granulated Erythritol (or preferred granulated sweetener)
- 8 oz (1 Cup) Unsweetened Applesauce
- 1 Tsp Pure Madagascar Bourbon Vanilla Extract
- ¾ Cup Unsweetened Non-Dairy Milk
- 2 Cups Powdered Erythritol (or preferred powdered sweetener)

Instructions

1. Preheat the oven to 425°F.

2. In a large mixing bowl, combine the coconut flour, arrowroot, baking powder, and granulated sweetener together, mix.

3. Now add the applesauce, vanilla, and milk. Mix again until you have a thick doughnut batter.

4. Grease a 12-count mini donut pan and spoon 1 tablespoon of doughnut batter into each of the 12 molds.

5. Bake the doughnuts for 8 minutes, remove and flip out onto a wire rack.

6. Repeat this process for the rest of the batter (about 2 ½ batches total)

7. To powder coat the baked doughnuts, place the powdered sweetener into a brown paper bag and in batches of about 6 doughnuts, place them into the powder, shake well to coat, take out and set on a wire rack. Add more powdered sweetener if needed between batches.

39. Healthy Homemade Vegan Doritos "Nacho Cheese"
Flavor (Gluten-Free, Allergy-Free)
Prep Time: 5 minutes

Cook Time: 10 minutes

Total Time: 15 minutes

Servings: 72

Ingredients

- 12 Mini Street-Style Corn Tortillas
- Coconut Oil Spray
- Nacho Cheese Powder:
- ⅓ Cup Nutritional Yeast
- 1 Tsp Chili Powder
- ½ Tsp Smoked Paprika
- ½ Tsp Paprika
- ¼ Tsp Garlic Powder
- ¼ Tsp Onion Powder
- Chipotle Powder (to taste, optional)
- ½ Tsp Tomato Powder (optional)
- Salt (to taste, optional)

Instructions

1. Preheat the oven to 350°F.

2. Stack your 12 mini tortillas and use a sharp knife to cut them (3 times) to make 6 triangles per tortilla (You'll end up with a total of 72 mini triangles).

3. Line 2 baking sheets with parchment paper or Silpats and space out your cut chips in a single layer on the sheets.

4. Spray the chips with the coconut oil and bake in the oven for 5-7 until slightly golden brown.

5. Remove the chips and flip them over, spray the newly flipped slide of the chips with the coconut oil and bake again for about 5 minutes until golden.

6. To make the nacho cheese powder, simply mix the spices together in a large bowl.

7. Once the chips are done baking, in batches, lightly spray both sides with the coconut oil and toss in the nacho cheese powder.

8. Remove the coated chips and set aside to cool.

9. Store the cooled finished chips in an airtight
   container or storage bags.